Type 2 Diabetes Log Book

Big Print Blood Glucose and Insulin Record Book

Date	Insulin Injections				Blood Glucose Reading								Notes
	Units Given				Breakfast		Lunch		Dinner		Before Bed		
	Breakfast	Lunch	Dinner	Bedtime	Before	After	Before	After	Before	After	Before	After	changes etc.
Monday													
Tuesday													
Wednesday													
Thursday													
Friday													
Saturday													
Sunday													

Vincent Van Gouache

Berhampore Press

BerhamporePress@gmail.com

ISBN-13:
978-1548542276

ISBN-10:
154854227X

Insulin Injections

Blood Glucose Readings

	Units Given				Breakfast		Lunch		Dinner		Before Bed		Notes
	Breakfast	Lunch	Dinner	Bedtime	Before	After	Before	After	Before	After	Before	After	Changes etc.
Monday													
Tuesday													
Wednesday													
Thursday													
Friday													
Saturday													
Sunday													

Insulin Injections

Blood Glucose Readings

	Units Given				Breakfast		Lunch		Dinner		Before Bed		Notes
	Breakfast	Lunch	Dinner	Bedtime	Before	After	Before	After	Before	After	Before	After	Changes etc.
Monday													
Tuesday													
Wednesday													
Thursday													
Friday													
Saturday													
Sunday													

Week Beginning

Insulin Injections

	Units Given			
	Breakfast	Lunch	Dinner	Bedtime
Monday				
Tuesday				
Wednesday				
Thursday				
Friday				
Saturday				
Sunday				

Blood Glucose Readings

	Breakfast		Lunch		Dinner		Before Bed		Notes
	Before	After	Before	After	Before	After	Before	After	Changes etc.
Monday									
Tuesday									
Wednesday									
Thursday									
Friday									
Saturday									
Sunday									

Week Beginning

Insulin Injections

	Units Given			
	Breakfast	Lunch	Dinner	Bedtime
Monday				
Tuesday				
Wednesday				
Thursday				
Friday				
Saturday				
Sunday				

Blood Glucose Readings

	Breakfast		Lunch		Dinner		Before Bed		Notes
	Before	After	Before	After	Before	After	Before	After	Changes etc.
Monday									
Tuesday									
Wednesday									
Thursday									
Friday									
Saturday									
Sunday									

Week Beginning

Insulin Injections

| | Units Given | | | | Blood Glucose Readings | | | | | | | | Notes |
| | Breakfast | Lunch | Dinner | Bedtime | Breakfast | | Lunch | | Dinner | | Before Bed | | Changes etc. |
					Before	After	Before	After	Before	After	Before	After	
Monday													
Tuesday													
Wednesday													
Thursday													
Friday													
Saturday													
Sunday													

Week Beginning

Insulin Injections

| | Units Given | | | | Blood Glucose Readings | | | | | | | | Notes |
| | Breakfast | Lunch | Dinner | Bedtime | Breakfast | | Lunch | | Dinner | | Before Bed | | Changes etc. |
					Before	After	Before	After	Before	After	Before	After	
Monday													
Tuesday													
Wednesday													
Thursday													
Friday													
Saturday													
Sunday													

Chart 1

Week Beginning

Insulin Injections

	Units Given		
	Breakfast	Lunch	Dinner	Bedtime
Monday				
Tuesday				
Wednesday				
Thursday				
Friday				
Saturday				
Sunday				

Blood Glucose Readings

	Breakfast		Lunch		Dinner		Before Bed		Notes
	Before	After	Before	After	Before	After	Before	After	Changes etc.
Monday									
Tuesday									
Wednesday									
Thursday									
Friday									
Saturday									
Sunday									

Chart 2

Week Beginning

Insulin Injections

	Units Given		
	Breakfast	Lunch	Dinner	Bedtime
Monday				
Tuesday				
Wednesday				
Thursday				
Friday				
Saturday				
Sunday				

Blood Glucose Readings

	Breakfast		Lunch		Dinner		Before Bed		Notes
	Before	After	Before	After	Before	After	Before	After	Changes etc.
Monday									
Tuesday									
Wednesday									
Thursday									
Friday									
Saturday									
Sunday									

Week Beginning

Insulin Injections

| | Units Given | | | | Blood Glucose Readings | | | | | | | | Notes |
| | Breakfast | Lunch | Dinner | Bedtime | Breakfast | | Lunch | | Dinner | | Before Bed | | Changes etc. |
					Before	After	Before	After	Before	After	Before	After	
Monday													
Tuesday													
Wednesday													
Thursday													
Friday													
Saturday													
Sunday													

Week Beginning

Insulin Injections

| | Units Given | | | | Blood Glucose Readings | | | | | | | | Notes |
| | Breakfast | Lunch | Dinner | Bedtime | Breakfast | | Lunch | | Dinner | | Before Bed | | Changes etc. |
					Before	After	Before	After	Before	After	Before	After	
Monday													
Tuesday													
Wednesday													
Thursday													
Friday													
Saturday													
Sunday													

Week Beginning

Insulin Injections
Blood Glucose Readings

| | Units Given | | | | Breakfast | | Lunch | | Dinner | | Before Bed | | Notes |
	Breakfast	Lunch	Dinner	Bedtime	Before	After	Before	After	Before	After	Before	After	Changes etc.
Monday													
Tuesday													
Wednesday													
Thursday													
Friday													
Saturday													
Sunday													

Week Beginning

Insulin Injections
Blood Glucose Readings

| | Units Given | | | | Breakfast | | Lunch | | Dinner | | Before Bed | | Notes |
	Breakfast	Lunch	Dinner	Bedtime	Before	After	Before	After	Before	After	Before	After	Changes etc.
Monday													
Tuesday													
Wednesday													
Thursday													
Friday													
Saturday													
Sunday													

Week Beginning

Insulin Injections

| | Units Given | | | | Blood Glucose Readings | | | | | | | | Notes |
| | Breakfast | Lunch | Dinner | Bedtime | Breakfast | | Lunch | | Dinner | | Before Bed | | Changes etc |
					Before	After	Before	After	Before	After	Before	After	
Monday													
Tuesday													
Wednesday													
Thursday													
Friday													
Saturday													
Sunday													

Week Beginning

Insulin Injections

| | Units Given | | | | Blood Glucose Readings | | | | | | | | Notes |
| | Breakfast | Lunch | Dinner | Bedtime | Breakfast | | Lunch | | Dinner | | Before Bed | | Changes etc |
					Before	After	Before	After	Before	After	Before	After	
Monday													
Tuesday													
Wednesday													
Thursday													
Friday													
Saturday													
Sunday													

Week Beginning

Insulin Injections

	Units Given			Breakfast		Lunch		Dinner		Before Bed		Notes
	Breakfast	Lunch	Dinner	Bedtime	Before	After	Before	After	Before	After	Before	After	Changes etc.
Monday													
Tuesday													
Wednesday													
Thursday													
Friday													
Saturday													
Sunday													

Blood Glucose Readings

Week Beginning

Insulin Injections

	Units Given			Breakfast		Lunch		Dinner		Before Bed		Notes
	Breakfast	Lunch	Dinner	Bedtime	Before	After	Before	After	Before	After	Before	After	Changes etc.
Monday													
Tuesday													
Wednesday													
Thursday													
Friday													
Saturday													
Sunday													

Blood Glucose Readings

Table 1

Week Beginning

| | Insulin Injections — Units Given | | | | Blood Glucose Readings | | | | | | | | Notes |
	Breakfast	Lunch	Dinner	Bedtime	Breakfast Before	Breakfast After	Lunch Before	Lunch After	Dinner Before	Dinner After	Before Bed Before	Before Bed After	Changes etc.
Monday													
Tuesday													
Wednesday													
Thursday													
Friday													
Saturday													
Sunday													

Table 2

Week Beginning

| | Insulin Injections — Units Given | | | | Blood Glucose Readings | | | | | | | | Notes |
	Breakfast	Lunch	Dinner	Bedtime	Breakfast Before	Breakfast After	Lunch Before	Lunch After	Dinner Before	Dinner After	Before Bed Before	Before Bed After	Changes etc.
Monday													
Tuesday													
Wednesday													
Thursday													
Friday													
Saturday													
Sunday													

Week Beginning

| | Insulin Injections | | | | Blood Glucose Readings | | | | | | | | Notes |
| | Units Given | | | | Breakfast | | Lunch | | Dinner | | Before Bed | | |
	Breakfast	Lunch	Dinner	Bedtime	Before	After	Before	After	Before	After	Before	After	Changes etc.
Monday													
Tuesday													
Wednesday													
Thursday													
Friday													
Saturday													
Sunday													

Week Beginning

| | Insulin Injections | | | | Blood Glucose Readings | | | | | | | | Notes |
| | Units Given | | | | Breakfast | | Lunch | | Dinner | | Before Bed | | |
	Breakfast	Lunch	Dinner	Bedtime	Before	After	Before	After	Before	After	Before	After	Changes etc.
Monday													
Tuesday													
Wednesday													
Thursday													
Friday													
Saturday													
Sunday													

Week Beginning

Insulin Injections

| | Units Given | | | | Blood Glucose Readings | | | | | | | | Notes |
	Breakfast	Lunch	Dinner	Bedtime	Breakfast Before	Breakfast After	Lunch Before	Lunch After	Dinner Before	Dinner After	Before Bed Before	Before Bed After	Changes etc.
Monday													
Tuesday													
Wednesday													
Thursday													
Friday													
Saturday													
Sunday													

Week Beginning

Insulin Injections

| | Units Given | | | | Blood Glucose Readings | | | | | | | | Notes |
	Breakfast	Lunch	Dinner	Bedtime	Breakfast Before	Breakfast After	Lunch Before	Lunch After	Dinner Before	Dinner After	Before Bed Before	Before Bed After	Changes etc.
Monday													
Tuesday													
Wednesday													
Thursday													
Friday													
Saturday													
Sunday													

Week Beginning

Insulin Injections — Units Given | Blood Glucose Readings

	Breakfast	Lunch	Dinner	Bedtime	Breakfast Before	Breakfast After	Lunch Before	Lunch After	Dinner Before	Dinner After	Before Bed Before	Before Bed After	Notes (Changes etc.)
Monday													
Tuesday													
Wednesday													
Thursday													
Friday													
Saturday													
Sunday													

Week Beginning

Insulin Injections — Units Given | Blood Glucose Readings

	Breakfast	Lunch	Dinner	Bedtime	Breakfast Before	Breakfast After	Lunch Before	Lunch After	Dinner Before	Dinner After	Before Bed Before	Before Bed After	Notes (Changes etc.)
Monday													
Tuesday													
Wednesday													
Thursday													
Friday													
Saturday													
Sunday													

Week Beginning

Insulin Injections				Blood Glucose Readings								Notes
Units Given				Breakfast		Lunch		Dinner		Before Bed		
Breakfast	Lunch	Dinner	Bedtime	Before	After	Before	After	Before	After	Before	After	Changes etc.
Monday												
Tuesday												
Wednesday												
Thursday												
Friday												
Saturday												
Sunday												

Week Beginning

Insulin Injections				Blood Glucose Readings								Notes
Units Given				Breakfast		Lunch		Dinner		Before Bed		
Breakfast	Lunch	Dinner	Bedtime	Before	After	Before	After	Before	After	Before	After	Changes etc.
Monday												
Tuesday												
Wednesday												
Thursday												
Friday												
Saturday												
Sunday												

Week Beginning

Insulin Injections

	Units Given			Blood Glucose Readings									Notes
	Breakfast	Lunch	Dinner	Bedtime	Breakfast		Lunch		Dinner		Before Bed		Changes etc.
					Before	After	Before	After	Before	After	Before	After	
Monday													
Tuesday													
Wednesday													
Thursday													
Friday													
Saturday													
Sunday													

Week Beginning

Insulin Injections

	Units Given			Blood Glucose Readings									Notes
	Breakfast	Lunch	Dinner	Bedtime	Breakfast		Lunch		Dinner		Before Bed		Changes etc.
					Before	After	Before	After	Before	After	Before	After	
Monday													
Tuesday													
Wednesday													
Thursday													
Friday													
Saturday													
Sunday													

Week Beginning

	Insulin Injections				Blood Glucose Readings								Notes
	Units Given				Breakfast		Lunch		Dinner		Before Bed		Changes etc.
	Breakfast	Lunch	Dinner	Bedtime	Before	After	Before	After	Before	After	Before	After	
Monday													
Tuesday													
Wednesday													
Thursday													
Friday													
Saturday													
Sunday													

Week Beginning

	Insulin Injections				Blood Glucose Readings								Notes
	Units Given				Breakfast		Lunch		Dinner		Before Bed		Changes etc.
	Breakfast	Lunch	Dinner	Bedtime	Before	After	Before	After	Before	After	Before	After	
Monday													
Tuesday													
Wednesday													
Thursday													
Friday													
Saturday													
Sunday													

Week Beginning

Insulin Injections

	Units Given			Blood Glucose Readings								Notes
	Breakfast	Lunch	Dinner	Bedtime	Breakfast		Lunch		Dinner		Before Bed		Changes etc.
					Before	After	Before	After	Before	After	Before	After	
Monday													
Tuesday													
Wednesday													
Thursday													
Friday													
Saturday													
Sunday													

Week Beginning

Insulin Injections

	Units Given			Blood Glucose Readings								Notes
	Breakfast	Lunch	Dinner	Bedtime	Breakfast		Lunch		Dinner		Before Bed		Changes etc.
					Before	After	Before	After	Before	After	Before	After	
Monday													
Tuesday													
Wednesday													
Thursday													
Friday													
Saturday													
Sunday													

Week Beginning

| | Insulin Injections – Units Given | | | | Blood Glucose Readings | | | | | | | | Notes |
	Breakfast	Lunch	Dinner	Bedtime	Breakfast Before	Breakfast After	Lunch Before	Lunch After	Dinner Before	Dinner After	Before Bed Before	Before Bed After	Changes etc
Monday													
Tuesday													
Wednesday													
Thursday													
Friday													
Saturday													
Sunday													

Week Beginning

| | Insulin Injections – Units Given | | | | Blood Glucose Readings | | | | | | | | Notes |
	Breakfast	Lunch	Dinner	Bedtime	Breakfast Before	Breakfast After	Lunch Before	Lunch After	Dinner Before	Dinner After	Before Bed Before	Before Bed After	Changes etc
Monday													
Tuesday													
Wednesday													
Thursday													
Friday													
Saturday													
Sunday													

Week Beginning

Insulin Injections

| | Units Given | | | | Blood Glucose Readings | | | | | | | | Notes |
	Breakfast	Lunch	Dinner	Bedtime	Breakfast Before	Breakfast After	Lunch Before	Lunch After	Dinner Before	Dinner After	Before Bed Before	Before Bed After	Changes etc.
Monday													
Tuesday													
Wednesday													
Thursday													
Friday													
Saturday													
Sunday													

Week Beginning

Insulin Injections

| | Units Given | | | | Blood Glucose Readings | | | | | | | | Notes |
	Breakfast	Lunch	Dinner	Bedtime	Breakfast Before	Breakfast After	Lunch Before	Lunch After	Dinner Before	Dinner After	Before Bed Before	Before Bed After	Changes etc.
Monday													
Tuesday													
Wednesday													
Thursday													
Friday													
Saturday													
Sunday													

Week Beginning

Insulin Injections

| | Units Given | | | Blood Glucose Readings | | | | | | | | Notes |
	Breakfast	Lunch	Dinner	Bedtime	Breakfast		Lunch		Dinner		Before Bed		Changes etc.
					Before	After	Before	After	Before	After	Before	After	
Monday													
Tuesday													
Wednesday													
Thursday													
Friday													
Saturday													
Sunday													

Week Beginning

Insulin Injections

| | Units Given | | | Blood Glucose Readings | | | | | | | | Notes |
	Breakfast	Lunch	Dinner	Bedtime	Breakfast		Lunch		Dinner		Before Bed		Changes etc.
					Before	After	Before	After	Before	After	Before	After	
Monday													
Tuesday													
Wednesday													
Thursday													
Friday													
Saturday													
Sunday													

Chart 1

Week Beginning

| | Insulin Injections — Units Given | | | | Blood Glucose Readings | | | | | | | | Notes |
	Breakfast	Lunch	Dinner	Bedtime	Breakfast Before	Breakfast After	Lunch Before	Lunch After	Dinner Before	Dinner After	Before Bed Before	Before Bed After	Changes etc.
Monday													
Tuesday													
Wednesday													
Thursday													
Friday													
Saturday													
Sunday													

Chart 2

Week Beginning

| | Insulin Injections — Units Given | | | | Blood Glucose Readings | | | | | | | | Notes |
	Breakfast	Lunch	Dinner	Bedtime	Breakfast Before	Breakfast After	Lunch Before	Lunch After	Dinner Before	Dinner After	Before Bed Before	Before Bed After	Changes etc.
Monday													
Tuesday													
Wednesday													
Thursday													
Friday													
Saturday													
Sunday													

Week Beginning

| | Insulin Injections Units Given | | | | Blood Glucose Readings | | | | | | | | Notes |
	Breakfast	Lunch	Dinner	Bedtime	Breakfast Before	Breakfast After	Lunch Before	Lunch After	Dinner Before	Dinner After	Before Bed Before	Before Bed After	Changes etc.
Monday													
Tuesday													
Wednesday													
Thursday													
Friday													
Saturday													
Sunday													

Week Beginning

| | Insulin Injections Units Given | | | | Blood Glucose Readings | | | | | | | | Notes |
	Breakfast	Lunch	Dinner	Bedtime	Breakfast Before	Breakfast After	Lunch Before	Lunch After	Dinner Before	Dinner After	Before Bed Before	Before Bed After	Changes etc.
Monday													
Tuesday													
Wednesday													
Thursday													
Friday													
Saturday													
Sunday													

Week Beginning

Insulin Injections

Blood Glucose Readings

	Units Given				Breakfast		Lunch		Dinner		Before Bed		Notes
	Breakfast	Lunch	Dinner	Bedtime	Before	After	Before	After	Before	After	Before	After	Changes etc.
Monday													
Tuesday													
Wednesday													
Thursday													
Friday													
Saturday													
Sunday													

Week Beginning

Insulin Injections

Blood Glucose Readings

	Units Given				Breakfast		Lunch		Dinner		Before Bed		Notes
	Breakfast	Lunch	Dinner	Bedtime	Before	After	Before	After	Before	After	Before	After	Changes etc.
Monday													
Tuesday													
Wednesday													
Thursday													
Friday													
Saturday													
Sunday													

Week Beginning

	Insulin Injections				Blood Glucose Readings								Notes
	Units Given				Breakfast		Lunch		Dinner		Before Bed		Changes etc.
	Breakfast	Lunch	Dinner	Bedtime	Before	After	Before	After	Before	After	Before	After	
Monday													
Tuesday													
Wednesday													
Thursday													
Friday													
Saturday													
Sunday													

Week Beginning

	Insulin Injections				Blood Glucose Readings								Notes
	Units Given				Breakfast		Lunch		Dinner		Before Bed		Changes etc.
	Breakfast	Lunch	Dinner	Bedtime	Before	After	Before	After	Before	After	Before	After	
Monday													
Tuesday													
Wednesday													
Thursday													
Friday													
Saturday													
Sunday													

Week Beginning

Insulin Injections — Units Given | **Blood Glucose Readings**

	Breakfast	Lunch	Dinner	Bedtime	Breakfast Before	Breakfast After	Lunch Before	Lunch After	Dinner Before	Dinner After	Before Bed Before	Before Bed After	Notes (Changes etc.)
Monday													
Tuesday													
Wednesday													
Thursday													
Friday													
Saturday													
Sunday													

Week Beginning

Insulin Injections — Units Given | **Blood Glucose Readings**

	Breakfast	Lunch	Dinner	Bedtime	Breakfast Before	Breakfast After	Lunch Before	Lunch After	Dinner Before	Dinner After	Before Bed Before	Before Bed After	Notes (Changes etc.)
Monday													
Tuesday													
Wednesday													
Thursday													
Friday													
Saturday													
Sunday													

Week Beginning

Insulin Injections				Blood Glucose Readings								Notes
Units Given				Breakfast		Lunch		Dinner		Before Bed		
Breakfast	Lunch	Dinner	Bedtime	Before	After	Before	After	Before	After	Before	After	Changes etc.
Monday												
Tuesday												
Wednesday												
Thursday												
Friday												
Saturday												
Sunday												

Week Beginning

Insulin Injections				Blood Glucose Readings								Notes
Units Given				Breakfast		Lunch		Dinner		Before Bed		
Breakfast	Lunch	Dinner	Bedtime	Before	After	Before	After	Before	After	Before	After	Changes etc.
Monday												
Tuesday												
Wednesday												
Thursday												
Friday												
Saturday												
Sunday												

Week Beginning

Insulin Injections — Units Given | **Blood Glucose Readings**

	Breakfast	Lunch	Dinner	Bedtime	Breakfast Before	Breakfast After	Lunch Before	Lunch After	Dinner Before	Dinner After	Before Bed Before	Before Bed After	Notes (Changes etc.)
Monday													
Tuesday													
Wednesday													
Thursday													
Friday													
Saturday													
Sunday													

Week Beginning

Insulin Injections — Units Given | **Blood Glucose Readings**

	Breakfast	Lunch	Dinner	Bedtime	Breakfast Before	Breakfast After	Lunch Before	Lunch After	Dinner Before	Dinner After	Before Bed Before	Before Bed After	Notes (Changes etc.)
Monday													
Tuesday													
Wednesday													
Thursday													
Friday													
Saturday													
Sunday													

Week Beginning

Insulin Injections

	Units Given				Blood Glucose Readings								
	Breakfast	Lunch	Dinner	Bedtime	Breakfast		Lunch		Dinner		Before Bed		Notes
					Before	After	Before	After	Before	After	Before	After	Changes etc
Monday													
Tuesday													
Wednesday													
Thursday													
Friday													
Saturday													
Sunday													

Week Beginning

Insulin Injections

	Units Given				Blood Glucose Readings								
	Breakfast	Lunch	Dinner	Bedtime	Breakfast		Lunch		Dinner		Before Bed		Notes
					Before	After	Before	After	Before	After	Before	After	Changes etc
Monday													
Tuesday													
Wednesday													
Thursday													
Friday													
Saturday													
Sunday													

Week Beginning

Insulin Injections

| | Units Given | | | | Blood Glucose Readings | | | | | | | | |
| | Breakfast | Lunch | Dinner | Bedtime | Breakfast | | Lunch | | Dinner | | Before Bed | | Notes |
					Before	After	Before	After	Before	After	Before	After	Changes etc.
Monday													
Tuesday													
Wednesday													
Thursday													
Friday													
Saturday													
Sunday													

Week Beginning

Insulin Injections

| | Units Given | | | | Blood Glucose Readings | | | | | | | | |
| | Breakfast | Lunch | Dinner | Bedtime | Breakfast | | Lunch | | Dinner | | Before Bed | | Notes |
					Before	After	Before	After	Before	After	Before	After	Changes etc.
Monday													
Tuesday													
Wednesday													
Thursday													
Friday													
Saturday													
Sunday													

Table 1

Week Beginning

| | Insulin Injections — Units Given | | | | Blood Glucose Readings | | | | | | | | Notes |
	Breakfast	Lunch	Dinner	Bedtime	Breakfast Before	Breakfast After	Lunch Before	Lunch After	Dinner Before	Dinner After	Before Bed Before	Before Bed After	Changes etc.
Monday													
Tuesday													
Wednesday													
Thursday													
Friday													
Saturday													
Sunday													

Table 2

Week Beginning

| | Insulin Injections — Units Given | | | | Blood Glucose Readings | | | | | | | | Notes |
	Breakfast	Lunch	Dinner	Bedtime	Breakfast Before	Breakfast After	Lunch Before	Lunch After	Dinner Before	Dinner After	Before Bed Before	Before Bed After	Changes etc.
Monday													
Tuesday													
Wednesday													
Thursday													
Friday													
Saturday													
Sunday													

Week Beginning

Insulin Injections

Blood Glucose Readings

	Units Given				Breakfast		Lunch		Dinner		Before Bed		Notes
	Breakfast	Lunch	Dinner	Bedtime	Before	After	Before	After	Before	After	Before	After	Changes etc.
Monday													
Tuesday													
Wednesday													
Thursday													
Friday													
Saturday													
Sunday													

Week Beginning

Insulin Injections

Blood Glucose Readings

	Units Given				Breakfast		Lunch		Dinner		Before Bed		Notes
	Breakfast	Lunch	Dinner	Bedtime	Before	After	Before	After	Before	After	Before	After	Changes etc.
Monday													
Tuesday													
Wednesday													
Thursday													
Friday													
Saturday													
Sunday													

Week Beginning

| | Insulin Injections Units Given | | | | Blood Glucose Readings | | | | | | | | Notes |
	Breakfast	Lunch	Dinner	Bedtime	Breakfast Before	Breakfast After	Lunch Before	Lunch After	Dinner Before	Dinner After	Before Bed Before	Before Bed After	Changes etc.
Monday													
Tuesday													
Wednesday													
Thursday													
Friday													
Saturday													
Sunday													

Week Beginning

| | Insulin Injections Units Given | | | | Blood Glucose Readings | | | | | | | | Notes |
	Breakfast	Lunch	Dinner	Bedtime	Breakfast Before	Breakfast After	Lunch Before	Lunch After	Dinner Before	Dinner After	Before Bed Before	Before Bed After	Changes etc.
Monday													
Tuesday													
Wednesday													
Thursday													
Friday													
Saturday													
Sunday													

Week Beginning _____

Insulin Injections / Blood Glucose Readings

	Units Given				Breakfast		Lunch		Dinner		Before Bed		Notes
	Breakfast	Lunch	Dinner	Bedtime	Before	After	Before	After	Before	After	Before	After	Changes etc.
Monday													
Tuesday													
Wednesday													
Thursday													
Friday													
Saturday													
Sunday													

Week Beginning _____

Insulin Injections / Blood Glucose Readings

	Units Given				Breakfast		Lunch		Dinner		Before Bed		Notes
	Breakfast	Lunch	Dinner	Bedtime	Before	After	Before	After	Before	After	Before	After	Changes etc.
Monday													
Tuesday													
Wednesday													
Thursday													
Friday													
Saturday													
Sunday													

Week Beginning

Insulin Injections

	Units Given				Blood Glucose Readings								Notes
	Breakfast	Lunch	Dinner	Bedtime	Breakfast		Lunch		Dinner		Before Bed		Changes etc.
					Before	After	Before	After	Before	After	Before	After	
Monday													
Tuesday													
Wednesday													
Thursday													
Friday													
Saturday													
Sunday													

Week Beginning

Insulin Injections

	Units Given				Blood Glucose Readings								Notes
	Breakfast	Lunch	Dinner	Bedtime	Breakfast		Lunch		Dinner		Before Bed		Changes etc.
					Before	After	Before	After	Before	After	Before	After	
Monday													
Tuesday													
Wednesday													
Thursday													
Friday													
Saturday													
Sunday													

Table 1

Week Beginning	Insulin Injections				Blood Glucose Readings								Notes
	Units Given				Breakfast		Lunch		Dinner		Before Bed		
	Breakfast	Lunch	Dinner	Bedtime	Before	After	Before	After	Before	After	Before	After	Changes etc.
Monday													
Tuesday													
Wednesday													
Thursday													
Friday													
Saturday													
Sunday													

Table 2

Week Beginning	Insulin Injections				Blood Glucose Readings								Notes
	Units Given				Breakfast		Lunch		Dinner		Before Bed		
	Breakfast	Lunch	Dinner	Bedtime	Before	After	Before	After	Before	After	Before	After	Changes etc.
Monday													
Tuesday													
Wednesday													
Thursday													
Friday													
Saturday													
Sunday													

Week Beginning

	Insulin Injections — Units Given				Blood Glucose Readings								Notes
					Breakfast		Lunch		Dinner		Before Bed		
	Breakfast	Lunch	Dinner	Bedtime	Before	After	Before	After	Before	After	Before	After	Changes etc.
Monday													
Tuesday													
Wednesday													
Thursday													
Friday													
Saturday													
Sunday													

Week Beginning

	Insulin Injections — Units Given				Blood Glucose Readings								Notes
					Breakfast		Lunch		Dinner		Before Bed		
	Breakfast	Lunch	Dinner	Bedtime	Before	After	Before	After	Before	After	Before	After	Changes etc.
Monday													
Tuesday													
Wednesday													
Thursday													
Friday													
Saturday													
Sunday													

Blood Glucose Readings (chart 1)

Week Beginning	Insulin Injections				Breakfast		Lunch		Dinner		Before Bed		Notes
	Units Given				Before	After	Before	After	Before	After	Before	After	Changes etc.
	Breakfast	Lunch	Dinner	Bedtime									
Monday													
Tuesday													
Wednesday													
Thursday													
Friday													
Saturday													
Sunday													

Blood Glucose Readings (chart 2)

Week Beginning	Insulin Injections				Breakfast		Lunch		Dinner		Before Bed		Notes
	Units Given				Before	After	Before	After	Before	After	Before	After	Changes etc.
	Breakfast	Lunch	Dinner	Bedtime									
Monday													
Tuesday													
Wednesday													
Thursday													
Friday													
Saturday													
Sunday													

Table 1

Week Beginning	Insulin Injections — Units Given				Blood Glucose Readings								Notes
	Breakfast	Lunch	Dinner	Bedtime	Breakfast Before	Breakfast After	Lunch Before	Lunch After	Dinner Before	Dinner After	Before Bed Before	Before Bed After	Changes etc.
Monday													
Tuesday													
Wednesday													
Thursday													
Friday													
Saturday													
Sunday													

Table 2

Week Beginning	Insulin Injections — Units Given				Blood Glucose Readings								Notes
	Breakfast	Lunch	Dinner	Bedtime	Breakfast Before	Breakfast After	Lunch Before	Lunch After	Dinner Before	Dinner After	Before Bed Before	Before Bed After	Changes etc.
Monday													
Tuesday													
Wednesday													
Thursday													
Friday													
Saturday													
Sunday													

Week Beginning

Insulin Injections

| | Units Given | | | | Blood Glucose Readings | | | | | | | | Notes |
	Breakfast	Lunch	Dinner	Bedtime	Breakfast Before	Breakfast After	Lunch Before	Lunch After	Dinner Before	Dinner After	Before Bed Before	Before Bed After	Changes etc.
Monday													
Tuesday													
Wednesday													
Thursday													
Friday													
Saturday													
Sunday													

Week Beginning

Insulin Injections

| | Units Given | | | | Blood Glucose Readings | | | | | | | | Notes |
	Breakfast	Lunch	Dinner	Bedtime	Breakfast Before	Breakfast After	Lunch Before	Lunch After	Dinner Before	Dinner After	Before Bed Before	Before Bed After	Changes etc.
Monday													
Tuesday													
Wednesday													
Thursday													
Friday													
Saturday													
Sunday													

Week Beginning

| | Insulin Injections
Units Given | | | | Blood Glucose Readings | | | | | | | | Notes |
| | Breakfast | Lunch | Dinner | Bedtime | Breakfast | | Lunch | | Dinner | | Before Bed | | Changes etc. |
					Before	After	Before	After	Before	After	Before	After	
Monday													
Tuesday													
Wednesday													
Thursday													
Friday													
Saturday													
Sunday													

Week Beginning

| | Insulin Injections
Units Given | | | | Blood Glucose Readings | | | | | | | | Notes |
| | Breakfast | Lunch | Dinner | Bedtime | Breakfast | | Lunch | | Dinner | | Before Bed | | Changes etc. |
					Before	After	Before	After	Before	After	Before	After	
Monday													
Tuesday													
Wednesday													
Thursday													
Friday													
Saturday													
Sunday													

Week Beginning

Insulin Injections

	Units Given				Blood Glucose Readings								Notes
	Breakfast	Lunch	Dinner	Bedtime	Breakfast		Lunch		Dinner		Before Bed		Changes etc.
					Before	After	Before	After	Before	After	Before	After	
Monday													
Tuesday													
Wednesday													
Thursday													
Friday													
Saturday													
Sunday													

Week Beginning

Insulin Injections

	Units Given				Blood Glucose Readings								Notes
	Breakfast	Lunch	Dinner	Bedtime	Breakfast		Lunch		Dinner		Before Bed		Changes etc.
					Before	After	Before	After	Before	After	Before	After	
Monday													
Tuesday													
Wednesday													
Thursday													
Friday													
Saturday													
Sunday													

Week Beginning

Insulin Injections

	Units Given				Blood Glucose Readings								Notes
	Breakfast	Lunch	Dinner	Bedtime	Breakfast		Lunch		Dinner		Before Bed		Changes etc.
					Before	After	Before	After	Before	After	Before	After	
Monday													
Tuesday													
Wednesday													
Thursday													
Friday													
Saturday													
Sunday													

Week Beginning

Insulin Injections

	Units Given				Blood Glucose Readings								Notes
	Breakfast	Lunch	Dinner	Bedtime	Breakfast		Lunch		Dinner		Before Bed		Changes etc.
					Before	After	Before	After	Before	After	Before	After	
Monday													
Tuesday													
Wednesday													
Thursday													
Friday													
Saturday													
Sunday													

Week Beginning

Insulin Injections					Blood Glucose Readings								
	Units Given				Breakfast		Lunch		Dinner		Before Bed		Notes
	Breakfast	Lunch	Dinner	Bedtime	Before	After	Before	After	Before	After	Before	After	Changes etc.
Monday													
Tuesday													
Wednesday													
Thursday													
Friday													
Saturday													
Sunday													

Week Beginning

Insulin Injections					Blood Glucose Readings								
	Units Given				Breakfast		Lunch		Dinner		Before Bed		Notes
	Breakfast	Lunch	Dinner	Bedtime	Before	After	Before	After	Before	After	Before	After	Changes etc.
Monday													
Tuesday													
Wednesday													
Thursday													
Friday													
Saturday													
Sunday													

Week Beginning

	Insulin Injections				Blood Glucose Readings								Notes
	Units Given				Breakfast		Lunch		Dinner		Before Bed		
	Breakfast	Lunch	Dinner	Bedtime	Before	After	Before	After	Before	After	Before	After	Changes etc.
Monday													
Tuesday													
Wednesday													
Thursday													
Friday													
Saturday													
Sunday													

Week Beginning

	Insulin Injections				Blood Glucose Readings								Notes
	Units Given				Breakfast		Lunch		Dinner		Before Bed		
	Breakfast	Lunch	Dinner	Bedtime	Before	After	Before	After	Before	After	Before	After	Changes etc.
Monday													
Tuesday													
Wednesday													
Thursday													
Friday													
Saturday													
Sunday													

Blood Glucose Readings

Week Beginning

Insulin Injections	Units Given			Blood Glucose Readings	Breakfast		Lunch		Dinner		Before Bed		Notes
	Breakfast	Lunch	Dinner	Bedtime	Before	After	Before	After	Before	After	Before	After	Changes etc.
Monday													
Tuesday													
Wednesday													
Thursday													
Friday													
Saturday													
Sunday													

Blood Glucose Readings

Week Beginning

Insulin Injections	Units Given			Blood Glucose Readings	Breakfast		Lunch		Dinner		Before Bed		Notes
	Breakfast	Lunch	Dinner	Bedtime	Before	After	Before	After	Before	After	Before	After	Changes etc.
Monday													
Tuesday													
Wednesday													
Thursday													
Friday													
Saturday													
Sunday													

Table 1

Week Beginning	Insulin Injections				Blood Glucose Readings								Notes
	Units Given				Breakfast		Lunch		Dinner		Before Bed		Changes etc.
	Breakfast	Lunch	Dinner	Bedtime	Before	After	Before	After	Before	After	Before	After	
Monday													
Tuesday													
Wednesday													
Thursday													
Friday													
Saturday													
Sunday													

Table 2

Week Beginning	Insulin Injections				Blood Glucose Readings								Notes
	Units Given				Breakfast		Lunch		Dinner		Before Bed		Changes etc.
	Breakfast	Lunch	Dinner	Bedtime	Before	After	Before	After	Before	After	Before	After	
Monday													
Tuesday													
Wednesday													
Thursday													
Friday													
Saturday													
Sunday													

Week Beginning

Insulin Injections				Blood Glucose Readings								Notes
Units Given				Breakfast		Lunch		Dinner		Before Bed		
Breakfast	Lunch	Dinner	Bedtime	Before	After	Before	After	Before	After	Before	After	Changes etc.
Monday												
Tuesday												
Wednesday												
Thursday												
Friday												
Saturday												
Sunday												

Week Beginning

Insulin Injections				Blood Glucose Readings								Notes
Units Given				Breakfast		Lunch		Dinner		Before Bed		
Breakfast	Lunch	Dinner	Bedtime	Before	After	Before	After	Before	After	Before	After	Changes etc.
Monday												
Tuesday												
Wednesday												
Thursday												
Friday												
Saturday												
Sunday												

Week Beginning

Insulin Injections

	Units Given				Blood Glucose Readings								Notes
					Breakfast		Lunch		Dinner		Before Bed		
	Breakfast	Lunch	Dinner	Bedtime	Before	After	Before	After	Before	After	Before	After	Changes etc.
Monday													
Tuesday													
Wednesday													
Thursday													
Friday													
Saturday													
Sunday													

Week Beginning

Insulin Injections

	Units Given				Blood Glucose Readings								Notes
					Breakfast		Lunch		Dinner		Before Bed		
	Breakfast	Lunch	Dinner	Bedtime	Before	After	Before	After	Before	After	Before	After	Changes etc.
Monday													
Tuesday													
Wednesday													
Thursday													
Friday													
Saturday													
Sunday													

Week Beginning

Insulin Injections — Blood Glucose Readings

| | Insulin Injections — Units Given | | | | Blood Glucose Readings | | | | | | | | Notes |
| | Breakfast | Lunch | Dinner | Bedtime | Breakfast | | Lunch | | Dinner | | Before Bed | | Changes etc. |
					Before	After	Before	After	Before	After	Before	After	
Monday													
Tuesday													
Wednesday													
Thursday													
Friday													
Saturday													
Sunday													

Week Beginning

Insulin Injections — Blood Glucose Readings

| | Insulin Injections — Units Given | | | | Blood Glucose Readings | | | | | | | | Notes |
| | Breakfast | Lunch | Dinner | Bedtime | Breakfast | | Lunch | | Dinner | | Before Bed | | Changes etc. |
					Before	After	Before	After	Before	After	Before	After	
Monday													
Tuesday													
Wednesday													
Thursday													
Friday													
Saturday													
Sunday													

Week Beginning

	Insulin Injections			Blood Glucose Readings									Notes
	Units Given			Breakfast		Lunch		Dinner		Before Bed			
	Breakfast	Lunch	Dinner	Bedtime	Before	After	Before	After	Before	After	Before	After	Changes etc.
Monday													
Tuesday													
Wednesday													
Thursday													
Friday													
Saturday													
Sunday													

Week Beginning

	Insulin Injections			Blood Glucose Readings									Notes
	Units Given			Breakfast		Lunch		Dinner		Before Bed			
	Breakfast	Lunch	Dinner	Bedtime	Before	After	Before	After	Before	After	Before	After	Changes etc.
Monday													
Tuesday													
Wednesday													
Thursday													
Friday													
Saturday													
Sunday													

Week Beginning

Insulin Injections

	Units Given			Breakfast		Lunch		Dinner		Before Bed		Notes
	Breakfast	Lunch	Dinner	Bedtime	Before	After	Before	After	Before	After	Before	After	Changes etc.
Monday													
Tuesday													
Wednesday													
Thursday													
Friday													
Saturday													
Sunday													

Blood Glucose Readings

Week Beginning

Insulin Injections

	Units Given			Breakfast		Lunch		Dinner		Before Bed		Notes
	Breakfast	Lunch	Dinner	Bedtime	Before	After	Before	After	Before	After	Before	After	Changes etc.
Monday													
Tuesday													
Wednesday													
Thursday													
Friday													
Saturday													
Sunday													

Blood Glucose Readings

Week Beginning

Insulin Injections

	Units Given				Blood Glucose Readings								Notes
	Breakfast	Lunch	Dinner	Bedtime	Breakfast		Lunch		Dinner		Before Bed		Changes etc.
					Before	After	Before	After	Before	After	Before	After	
Monday													
Tuesday													
Wednesday													
Thursday													
Friday													
Saturday													
Sunday													

Week Beginning

Insulin Injections

	Units Given				Blood Glucose Readings								Notes
	Breakfast	Lunch	Dinner	Bedtime	Breakfast		Lunch		Dinner		Before Bed		Changes etc.
					Before	After	Before	After	Before	After	Before	After	
Monday													
Tuesday													
Wednesday													
Thursday													
Friday													
Saturday													
Sunday													

Table 1

Week Beginning

	Insulin Injections — Units Given				Blood Glucose Readings								Notes
					Breakfast		Lunch		Dinner		Before Bed		Changes etc.
	Breakfast	Lunch	Dinner	Bedtime	Before	After	Before	After	Before	After	Before	After	
Monday													
Tuesday													
Wednesday													
Thursday													
Friday													
Saturday													
Sunday													

Table 2

Week Beginning

	Insulin Injections — Units Given				Blood Glucose Readings								Notes
					Breakfast		Lunch		Dinner		Before Bed		Changes etc.
	Breakfast	Lunch	Dinner	Bedtime	Before	After	Before	After	Before	After	Before	After	
Monday													
Tuesday													
Wednesday													
Thursday													
Friday													
Saturday													
Sunday													

Week Beginning

	Insulin Injections				Blood Glucose Readings								
	Units Given				Breakfast		Lunch		Dinner		Before Bed		Notes
	Breakfast	Lunch	Dinner	Bedtime	Before	After	Before	After	Before	After	Before	After	Changes etc.
Monday													
Tuesday													
Wednesday													
Thursday													
Friday													
Saturday													
Sunday													

Week Beginning

	Insulin Injections				Blood Glucose Readings								
	Units Given				Breakfast		Lunch		Dinner		Before Bed		Notes
	Breakfast	Lunch	Dinner	Bedtime	Before	After	Before	After	Before	After	Before	After	Changes etc.
Monday													
Tuesday													
Wednesday													
Thursday													
Friday													
Saturday													
Sunday													

Table 1

Week Beginning	Insulin Injections				Blood Glucose Readings								Notes
	Units Given				Breakfast		Lunch		Dinner		Before Bed		
	Breakfast	Lunch	Dinner	Bedtime	Before	After	Before	After	Before	After	Before	After	Changes etc.
Monday													
Tuesday													
Wednesday													
Thursday													
Friday													
Saturday													
Sunday													

Table 2

Week Beginning	Insulin Injections				Blood Glucose Readings								Notes
	Units Given				Breakfast		Lunch		Dinner		Before Bed		
	Breakfast	Lunch	Dinner	Bedtime	Before	After	Before	After	Before	After	Before	After	Changes etc.
Monday													
Tuesday													
Wednesday													
Thursday													
Friday													
Saturday													
Sunday													

Week Beginning

	Insulin Injections – Units Given				Blood Glucose Readings								Notes
	Breakfast	Lunch	Dinner	Bedtime	Breakfast Before	Breakfast After	Lunch Before	Lunch After	Dinner Before	Dinner After	Before Bed Before	Before Bed After	Changes etc.
Monday													
Tuesday													
Wednesday													
Thursday													
Friday													
Saturday													
Sunday													

Week Beginning

	Insulin Injections – Units Given				Blood Glucose Readings								Notes
	Breakfast	Lunch	Dinner	Bedtime	Breakfast Before	Breakfast After	Lunch Before	Lunch After	Dinner Before	Dinner After	Before Bed Before	Before Bed After	Changes etc.
Monday													
Tuesday													
Wednesday													
Thursday													
Friday													
Saturday													
Sunday													

Week Beginning

| | Insulin Injections – Units Given | | | | Blood Glucose Readings | | | | | | | | Notes |
	Breakfast	Lunch	Dinner	Bedtime	Breakfast Before	Breakfast After	Lunch Before	Lunch After	Dinner Before	Dinner After	Before Bed Before	Before Bed After	Changes etc.
Monday													
Tuesday													
Wednesday													
Thursday													
Friday													
Saturday													
Sunday													

Week Beginning

| | Insulin Injections – Units Given | | | | Blood Glucose Readings | | | | | | | | Notes |
	Breakfast	Lunch	Dinner	Bedtime	Breakfast Before	Breakfast After	Lunch Before	Lunch After	Dinner Before	Dinner After	Before Bed Before	Before Bed After	Changes etc.
Monday													
Tuesday													
Wednesday													
Thursday													
Friday													
Saturday													
Sunday													

Table 1

Week Beginning	Insulin Injections				Blood Glucose Readings								Notes
	Units Given				Breakfast		Lunch		Dinner		Before Bed		
	Breakfast	Lunch	Dinner	Bedtime	Before	After	Before	After	Before	After	Before	After	Changes etc.
Monday													
Tuesday													
Wednesday													
Thursday													
Friday													
Saturday													
Sunday													

Table 2

Week Beginning	Insulin Injections				Blood Glucose Readings								Notes
	Units Given				Breakfast		Lunch		Dinner		Before Bed		
	Breakfast	Lunch	Dinner	Bedtime	Before	After	Before	After	Before	After	Before	After	Changes etc.
Monday													
Tuesday													
Wednesday													
Thursday													
Friday													
Saturday													
Sunday													

Week Beginning

Insulin Injections

	Units Given			Blood Glucose Readings								Notes
	Breakfast	Lunch	Dinner	Bedtime	Breakfast		Lunch		Dinner		Before Bed		Changes etc.
					Before	After	Before	After	Before	After	Before	After	
Monday													
Tuesday													
Wednesday													
Thursday													
Friday													
Saturday													
Sunday													

Week Beginning

Insulin Injections

	Units Given			Blood Glucose Readings								Notes
	Breakfast	Lunch	Dinner	Bedtime	Breakfast		Lunch		Dinner		Before Bed		Changes etc.
					Before	After	Before	After	Before	After	Before	After	
Monday													
Tuesday													
Wednesday													
Thursday													
Friday													
Saturday													
Sunday													

Week Beginning

	Insulin Injections – Units Given			Blood Glucose Readings								Notes
	Breakfast	Lunch	Dinner	Bedtime	Breakfast		Lunch		Dinner		Before Bed		Changes etc.
					Before	After	Before	After	Before	After	Before	After	
Monday													
Tuesday													
Wednesday													
Thursday													
Friday													
Saturday													
Sunday													

Week Beginning

	Insulin Injections – Units Given			Blood Glucose Readings								Notes
	Breakfast	Lunch	Dinner	Bedtime	Breakfast		Lunch		Dinner		Before Bed		Changes etc.
					Before	After	Before	After	Before	After	Before	After	
Monday													
Tuesday													
Wednesday													
Thursday													
Friday													
Saturday													
Sunday													

Week Beginning

Insulin Injections

| | Units Given | | | | Blood Glucose Readings | | | | | | | | Notes |
| | Breakfast | Lunch | Dinner | Bedtime | Breakfast | | Lunch | | Dinner | | Before Bed | | Changes etc. |
					Before	After	Before	After	Before	After	Before	After	
Monday													
Tuesday													
Wednesday													
Thursday													
Friday													
Saturday													
Sunday													

Week Beginning

Insulin Injections

| | Units Given | | | | Blood Glucose Readings | | | | | | | | Notes |
| | Breakfast | Lunch | Dinner | Bedtime | Breakfast | | Lunch | | Dinner | | Before Bed | | Changes etc. |
					Before	After	Before	After	Before	After	Before	After	
Monday													
Tuesday													
Wednesday													
Thursday													
Friday													
Saturday													
Sunday													

Week Beginning

Insulin Injections

| | Units Given | | | | Blood Glucose Readings | | | | | | | | | Notes |
| | Breakfast | Lunch | Dinner | Bedtime | Breakfast | | Lunch | | Dinner | | Before Bed | | Changes etc. |
					Before	After	Before	After	Before	After	Before	After	
Monday													
Tuesday													
Wednesday													
Thursday													
Friday													
Saturday													
Sunday													

Week Beginning

Insulin Injections

| | Units Given | | | | Blood Glucose Readings | | | | | | | | | Notes |
| | Breakfast | Lunch | Dinner | Bedtime | Breakfast | | Lunch | | Dinner | | Before Bed | | Changes etc. |
					Before	After	Before	After	Before	After	Before	After	
Monday													
Tuesday													
Wednesday													
Thursday													
Friday													
Saturday													
Sunday													

Insulin Injections / Blood Glucose Readings

Week Beginning

	Units Given				Breakfast		Lunch		Dinner		Before Bed		Notes
	Breakfast	Lunch	Dinner	Bedtime	Before	After	Before	After	Before	After	Before	After	Changes etc.
Monday													
Tuesday													
Wednesday													
Thursday													
Friday													
Saturday													
Sunday													

Insulin Injections / Blood Glucose Readings

Week Beginning

	Units Given				Breakfast		Lunch		Dinner		Before Bed		Notes
	Breakfast	Lunch	Dinner	Bedtime	Before	After	Before	After	Before	After	Before	After	Changes etc.
Monday													
Tuesday													
Wednesday													
Thursday													
Friday													
Saturday													
Sunday													

Week Beginning

Insulin Injections

	Units Given			Breakfast		Lunch		Dinner		Before Bed		Notes
	Breakfast	Lunch	Dinner	Bedtime	Before	After	Before	After	Before	After	Before	After	Changes etc.
Monday													
Tuesday													
Wednesday													
Thursday													
Friday													
Saturday													
Sunday													

Blood Glucose Readings

Week Beginning

Insulin Injections

	Units Given			Breakfast		Lunch		Dinner		Before Bed		Notes
	Breakfast	Lunch	Dinner	Bedtime	Before	After	Before	After	Before	After	Before	After	Changes etc.
Monday													
Tuesday													
Wednesday													
Thursday													
Friday													
Saturday													
Sunday													

Blood Glucose Readings

Week Beginning

Insulin Injections — **Blood Glucose Readings**

	Units Given				Breakfast		Lunch		Dinner		Before Bed		Notes
	Breakfast	Lunch	Dinner	Bedtime	Before	After	Before	After	Before	After	Before	After	Changes etc.
Monday													
Tuesday													
Wednesday													
Thursday													
Friday													
Saturday													
Sunday													

Week Beginning

Insulin Injections — **Blood Glucose Readings**

	Units Given				Breakfast		Lunch		Dinner		Before Bed		Notes
	Breakfast	Lunch	Dinner	Bedtime	Before	After	Before	After	Before	After	Before	After	Changes etc.
Monday													
Tuesday													
Wednesday													
Thursday													
Friday													
Saturday													
Sunday													

Week Beginning

	Insulin Injections			Blood Glucose Readings								Notes
	Units Given			Breakfast		Lunch		Dinner		Before Bed		
	Breakfast	Lunch	Dinner	Bedtime	Before	After	Before	After	Before	After	Before	After	Changes etc.
Monday													
Tuesday													
Wednesday													
Thursday													
Friday													
Saturday													
Sunday													

Week Beginning

	Insulin Injections			Blood Glucose Readings								Notes
	Units Given			Breakfast		Lunch		Dinner		Before Bed		
	Breakfast	Lunch	Dinner	Bedtime	Before	After	Before	After	Before	After	Before	After	Changes etc.
Monday													
Tuesday													
Wednesday													
Thursday													
Friday													
Saturday													
Sunday													

Week Beginning

Insulin Injections

	Units Given				Blood Glucose Readings								Notes
	Breakfast	Lunch	Dinner	Bedtime	Breakfast Before	Breakfast After	Lunch Before	Lunch After	Dinner Before	Dinner After	Before Bed Before	Before Bed After	Changes etc.
Monday													
Tuesday													
Wednesday													
Thursday													
Friday													
Saturday													
Sunday													

Week Beginning

Insulin Injections

	Units Given				Blood Glucose Readings								Notes
	Breakfast	Lunch	Dinner	Bedtime	Breakfast Before	Breakfast After	Lunch Before	Lunch After	Dinner Before	Dinner After	Before Bed Before	Before Bed After	Changes etc.
Monday													
Tuesday													
Wednesday													
Thursday													
Friday													
Saturday													
Sunday													

Week Beginning

	Insulin Injections			Blood Glucose Readings									Notes
	Units Given			Breakfast		Lunch		Dinner		Before Bed			
	Breakfast	Lunch	Dinner	Bedtime	Before	After	Before	After	Before	After	Before	After	Changes etc.
Monday													
Tuesday													
Wednesday													
Thursday													
Friday													
Saturday													
Sunday													

Week Beginning

	Insulin Injections			Blood Glucose Readings									Notes
	Units Given			Breakfast		Lunch		Dinner		Before Bed			
	Breakfast	Lunch	Dinner	Bedtime	Before	After	Before	After	Before	After	Before	After	Changes etc.
Monday													
Tuesday													
Wednesday													
Thursday													
Friday													
Saturday													
Sunday													

Week Beginning

Insulin Injections

| | Units Given | | | Blood Glucose Readings | | | | | | | | Notes |
| | Breakfast | Lunch | Dinner | Bedtime | Breakfast | | Lunch | | Dinner | | Before Bed | | Changes etc. |
					Before	After	Before	After	Before	After	Before	After	
Monday													
Tuesday													
Wednesday													
Thursday													
Friday													
Saturday													
Sunday													

Week Beginning

Insulin Injections

| | Units Given | | | Blood Glucose Readings | | | | | | | | Notes |
| | Breakfast | Lunch | Dinner | Bedtime | Breakfast | | Lunch | | Dinner | | Before Bed | | Changes etc. |
					Before	After	Before	After	Before	After	Before	After	
Monday													
Tuesday													
Wednesday													
Thursday													
Friday													
Saturday													
Sunday													

Week Beginning

Insulin Injections

	Units Given				Blood Glucose Readings								Notes
	Breakfast	Lunch	Dinner	Bedtime	Breakfast		Lunch		Dinner		Before Bed		Changes etc.
					Before	After	Before	After	Before	After	Before	After	
Monday													
Tuesday													
Wednesday													
Thursday													
Friday													
Saturday													
Sunday													

Week Beginning

Insulin Injections

	Units Given				Blood Glucose Readings								Notes
	Breakfast	Lunch	Dinner	Bedtime	Breakfast		Lunch		Dinner		Before Bed		Changes etc.
					Before	After	Before	After	Before	After	Before	After	
Monday													
Tuesday													
Wednesday													
Thursday													
Friday													
Saturday													
Sunday													

Week Beginning

Insulin Injections

| | Units Given | | | | Blood Glucose Readings | | | | | | | | Notes |
	Breakfast	Lunch	Dinner	Bedtime	Breakfast		Lunch		Dinner		Before Bed		Changes etc.
					Before	After	Before	After	Before	After	Before	After	
Monday													
Tuesday													
Wednesday													
Thursday													
Friday													
Saturday													
Sunday													

Week Beginning

Insulin Injections

| | Units Given | | | | Blood Glucose Readings | | | | | | | | Notes |
	Breakfast	Lunch	Dinner	Bedtime	Breakfast		Lunch		Dinner		Before Bed		Changes etc.
					Before	After	Before	After	Before	After	Before	After	
Monday													
Tuesday													
Wednesday													
Thursday													
Friday													
Saturday													
Sunday													

Week Beginning

	Insulin Injections				Blood Glucose Readings								
	Units Given				Breakfast		Lunch		Dinner		Before Bed		Notes
	Breakfast	Lunch	Dinner	Bedtime	Before	After	Before	After	Before	After	Before	After	Changes etc.
Monday													
Tuesday													
Wednesday													
Thursday													
Friday													
Saturday													
Sunday													

Week Beginning

	Insulin Injections				Blood Glucose Readings								
	Units Given				Breakfast		Lunch		Dinner		Before Bed		Notes
	Breakfast	Lunch	Dinner	Bedtime	Before	After	Before	After	Before	After	Before	After	Changes etc.
Monday													
Tuesday													
Wednesday													
Thursday													
Friday													
Saturday													
Sunday													

Week Beginning

Insulin Injections

| | Units Given | | | | Blood Glucose Readings | | | | | | | | Notes |
| | Breakfast | Lunch | Dinner | Bedtime | Breakfast | | Lunch | | Dinner | | Before Bed | | Changes etc. |
					Before	After	Before	After	Before	After	Before	After	
Monday													
Tuesday													
Wednesday													
Thursday													
Friday													
Saturday													
Sunday													

Week Beginning

Insulin Injections

| | Units Given | | | | Blood Glucose Readings | | | | | | | | Notes |
| | Breakfast | Lunch | Dinner | Bedtime | Breakfast | | Lunch | | Dinner | | Before Bed | | Changes etc. |
					Before	After	Before	After	Before	After	Before	After	
Monday													
Tuesday													
Wednesday													
Thursday													
Friday													
Saturday													
Sunday													

Week Beginning

Insulin Injections

	Units Given				Blood Glucose Readings								Notes
	Breakfast	Lunch	Dinner	Bedtime	Breakfast		Lunch		Dinner		Before Bed		Changes etc.
					Before	After	Before	After	Before	After	Before	After	
Monday													
Tuesday													
Wednesday													
Thursday													
Friday													
Saturday													
Sunday													

Week Beginning

Insulin Injections

	Units Given				Blood Glucose Readings								Notes
	Breakfast	Lunch	Dinner	Bedtime	Breakfast		Lunch		Dinner		Before Bed		Changes etc.
					Before	After	Before	After	Before	After	Before	After	
Monday													
Tuesday													
Wednesday													
Thursday													
Friday													
Saturday													
Sunday													

Week Beginning

Insulin Injections

| | Units Given | | | | Breakfast | | Lunch | | Dinner | | Before Bed | | Notes |
	Breakfast	Lunch	Dinner	Bedtime	Before	After	Before	After	Before	After	Before	After	Changes etc.
Monday													
Tuesday													
Wednesday													
Thursday													
Friday													
Saturday													
Sunday													

Blood Glucose Readings

Week Beginning

Insulin Injections

| | Units Given | | | | Breakfast | | Lunch | | Dinner | | Before Bed | | Notes |
	Breakfast	Lunch	Dinner	Bedtime	Before	After	Before	After	Before	After	Before	After	Changes etc.
Monday													
Tuesday													
Wednesday													
Thursday													
Friday													
Saturday													
Sunday													

Blood Glucose Readings

Week Beginning

Insulin Injections

	Units Given				Blood Glucose Readings								Notes
	Breakfast	Lunch	Dinner	Bedtime	Breakfast		Lunch		Dinner		Before Bed		Changes etc.
					Before	After	Before	After	Before	After	Before	After	
Monday													
Tuesday													
Wednesday													
Thursday													
Friday													
Saturday													
Sunday													

Week Beginning

Insulin Injections

	Units Given				Blood Glucose Readings								Notes
	Breakfast	Lunch	Dinner	Bedtime	Breakfast		Lunch		Dinner		Before Bed		Changes etc.
					Before	After	Before	After	Before	After	Before	After	
Monday													
Tuesday													
Wednesday													
Thursday													
Friday													
Saturday													
Sunday													

Made in the USA
Coppell, TX
25 September 2020